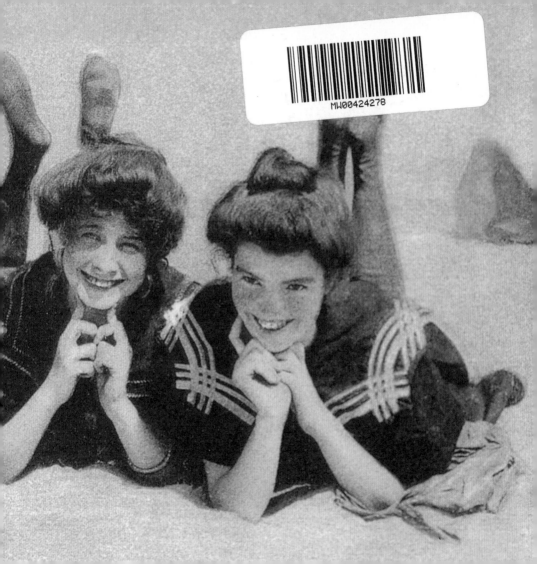

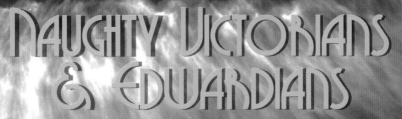

NAUGHTY VICTORIANS & EDWARDIANS

Early Images of Bathing Beauties

Mary L. Martin
Tina Skinner

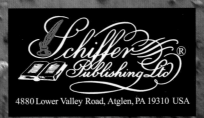

4880 Lower Valley Road, Atglen, PA 19310 USA

About the Authors

Mary Martin Postcards is a three-generation family business and the largest postcard operation in the world. In addition to a warehouse facility in Perryville, Maryland, the company is a presence at postcard shows worldwide, and produces many shows, including the nation's largest postcard show in York, Pennsylvania, in November. They are located at www.marylmartin.com and can be telephoned at 410-642-3581. Tina Skinner is a professional writer and editor.

Published by Schiffer Publishing Ltd.
4880 Lower Valley Road
Atglen, PA 19310
Phone: (610) 593-1777; Fax: (610) 593-2002
E-mail: Info@schifferbooks.com

For the largest selection of fine reference books on this
and related subjects, please visit our web site at
www.schifferbooks.com
We are always looking for people to write books on new
and related subjects. If you have an idea for a book
please contact us at the above address.

This book may be purchased from the publisher.
Include $3.95 for shipping.
Please try your bookstore first.
You may write for a free catalog.

In Europe, Schiffer books are distributed by
Bushwood Books
6 Marksbury Ave.
Kew Gardens
Surrey TW9 4JF England
Phone: 44 (0) 20 8392-8585; Fax: 44 (0) 20 8392-9876
E-mail: info@bushwoodbooks.co.uk
Free postage in the U.K., Europe; air mail at cost.

Designed by John P. Cheek
Cover Design by John P. Cheek
Type set in Humanist 521 BT

ISBN: 0-7643-2115-3
Printed in China

Introduction

In the interests of sobriety, and prudence, and modesty, and whatever, beachgoers in the Victorian era segregated themselves according to gender. Women discretely prepared themselves for a dip in the saltwater by trundling out to sea in a wheeled dressing room, and emerging from the dry compartment into water roped off for females only. It was ever so proper, with clothing designed to cover nearly all flesh below the neck, along with caps to crown their hair. So who would think that a sexy thought ever penetrated all that fabric?

There's no hiding the bare truth, though. Join in as photographers unveil the feminine side of Victorian-era women, playfully exposing themselves to sun and film approximately 100 years ago. It's a charming romp through the holiday antics of men and women out simply enjoying themselves. Share in the fun, created for postcards that were widely disseminated at the turn of the century.

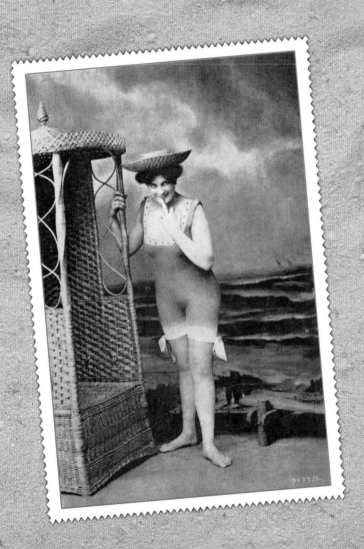

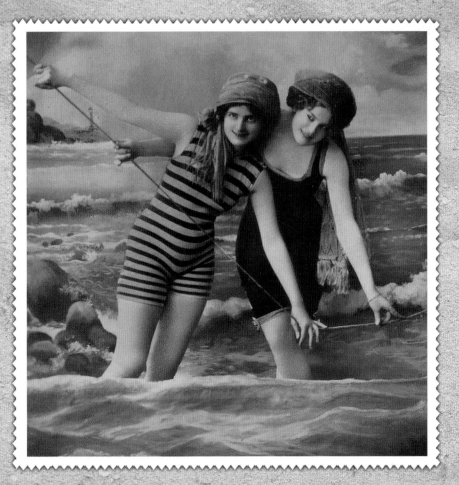

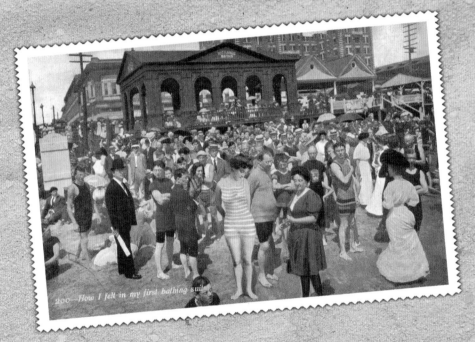

200—*How I felt in my first bathing suit*

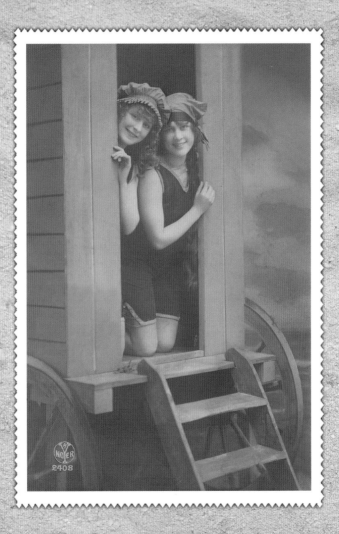

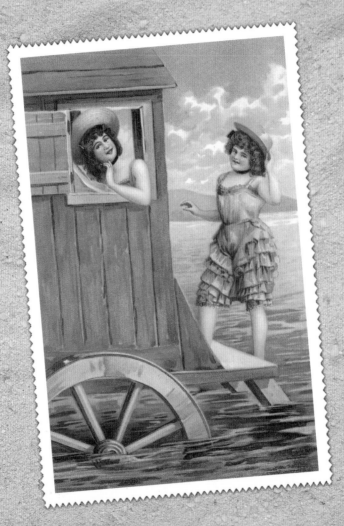

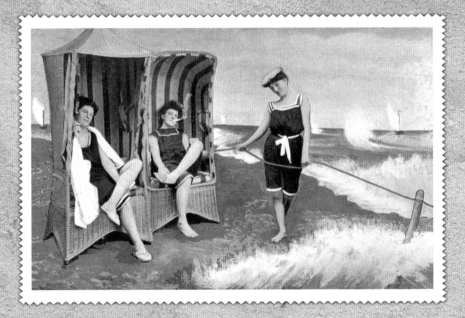

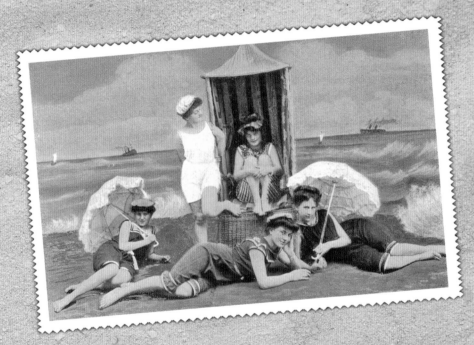

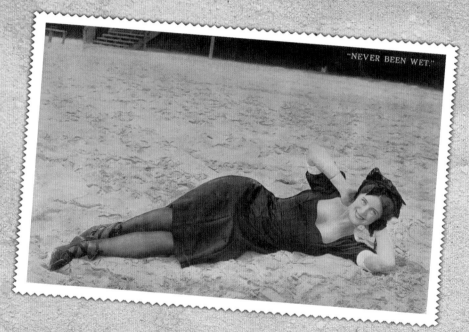

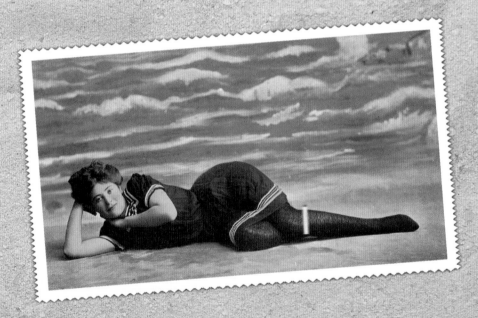

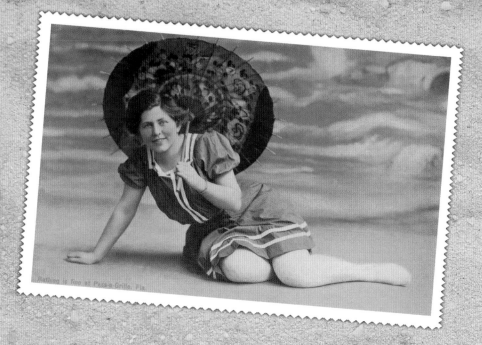

Bathing is fun at Pass-a-Grille, Fla.

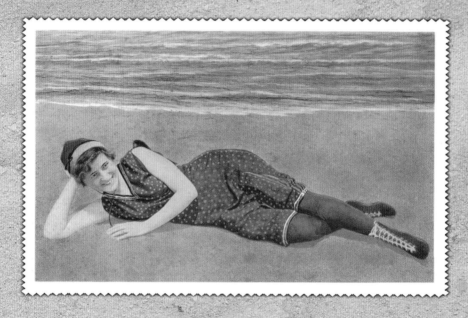

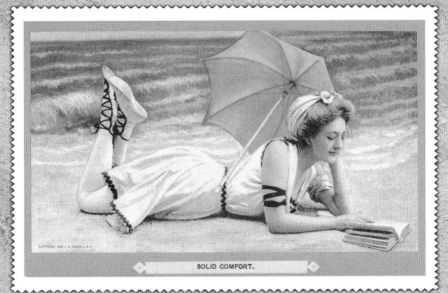

SOLID COMFORT.

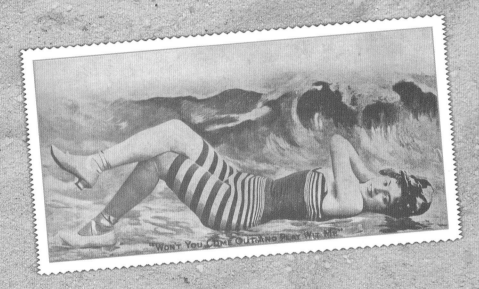

"WON'T YOU COME OUT AND PLAY WIT ME"

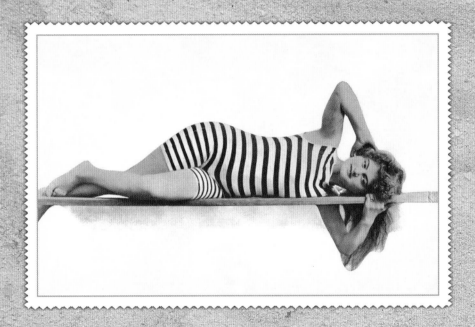

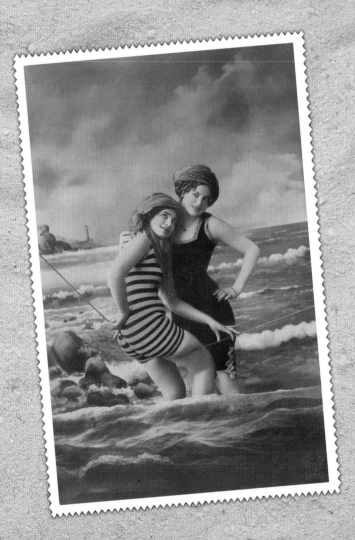

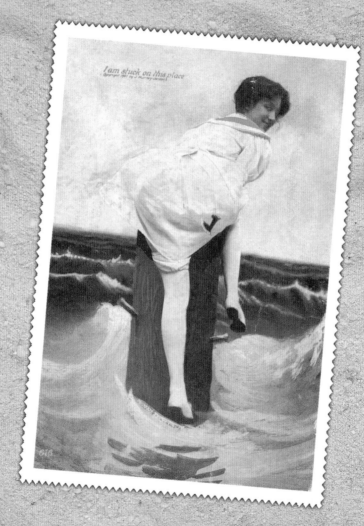

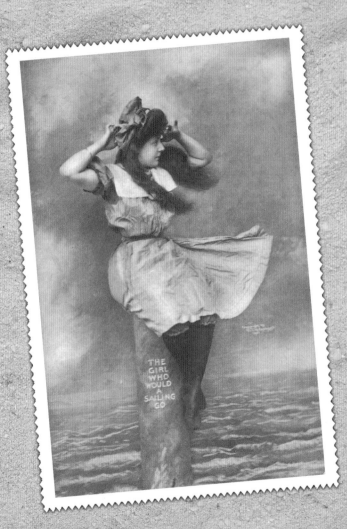

THE
GIRL
WHO
WOULD
A
SAILING
GO

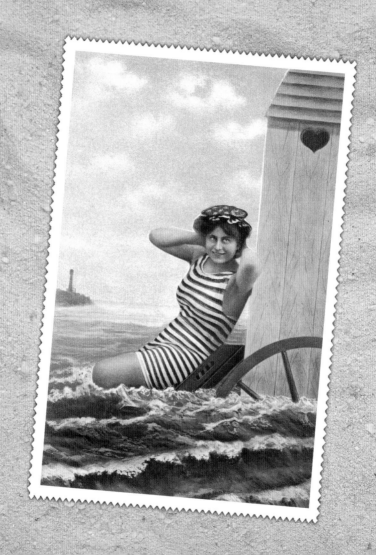

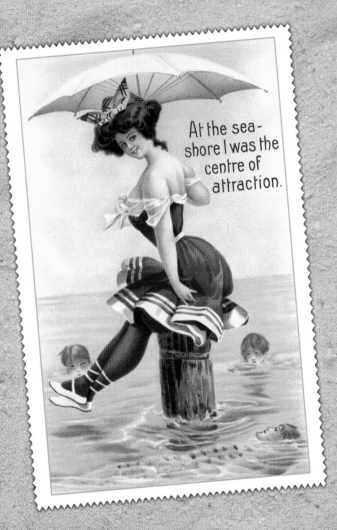

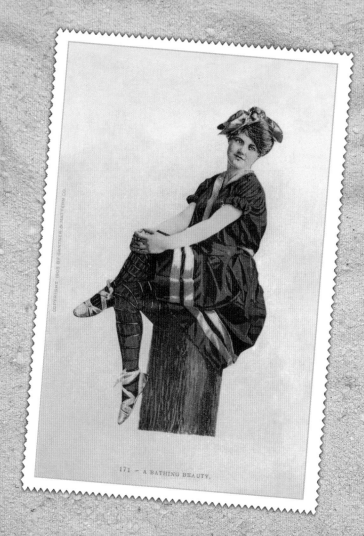

171 — A BATHING BEAUTY.

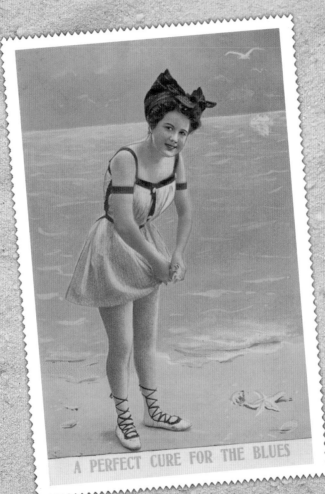

A PERFECT CURE FOR THE BLUES

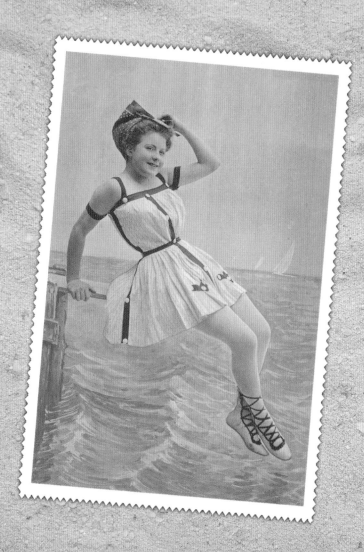

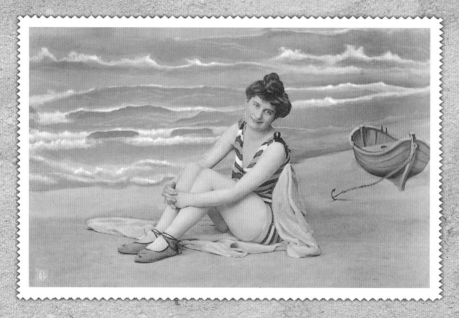

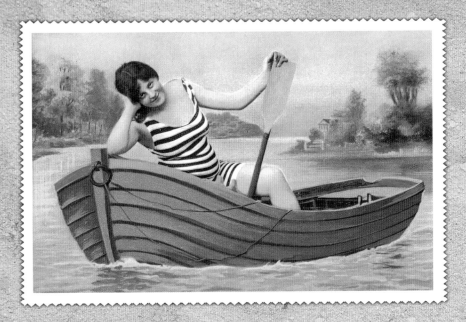

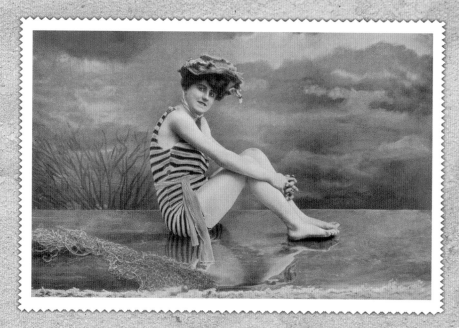

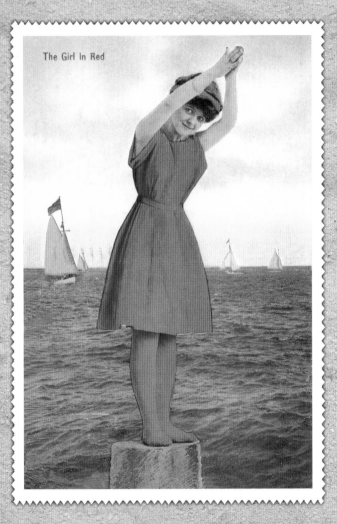

The Girl In Red

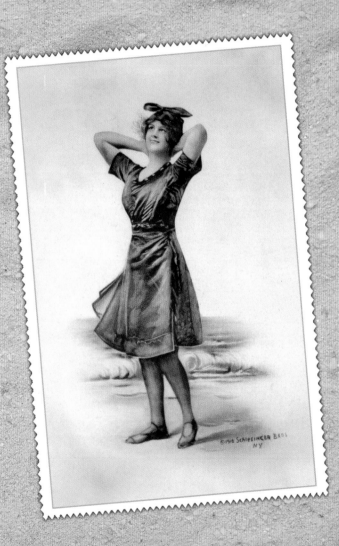

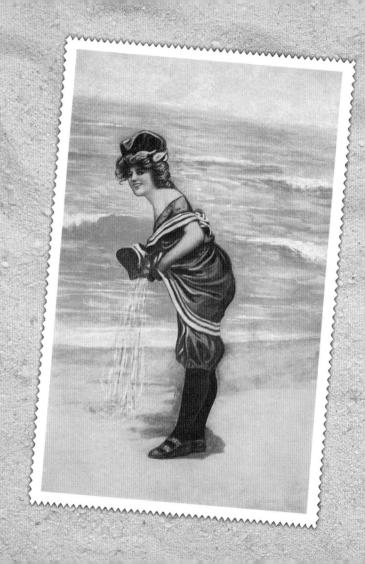

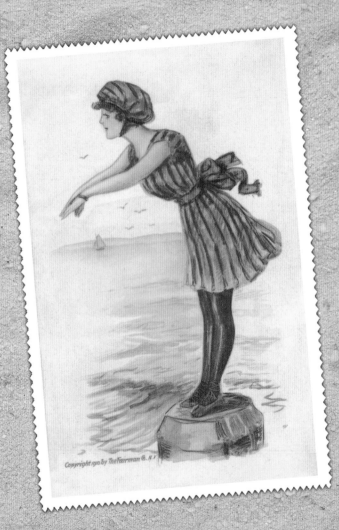

Copyright 1910 by The Fairman Co. N.Y.

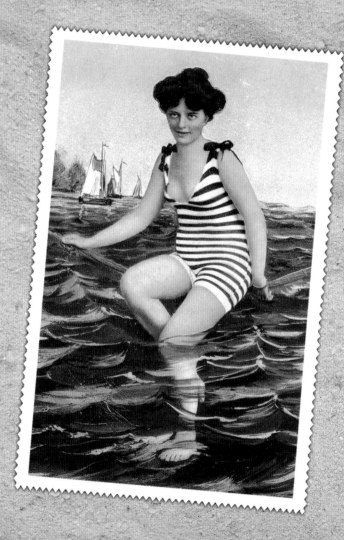

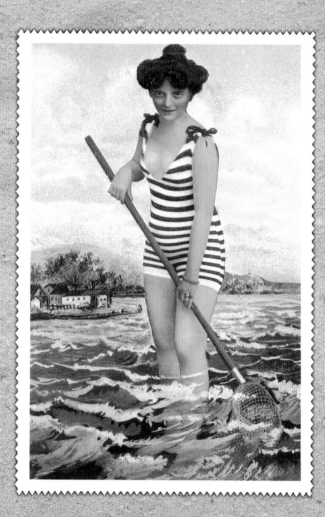

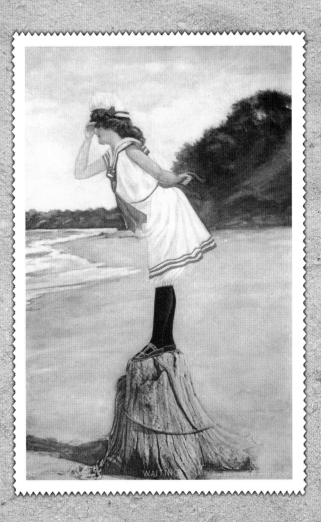

WAITING

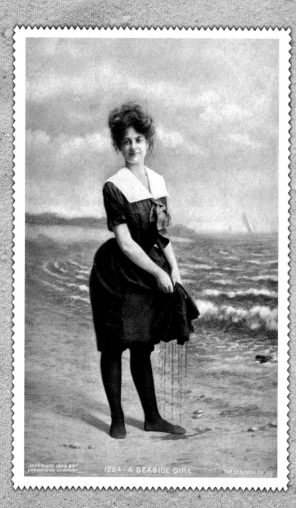

1284—A SEASIDE GIRL

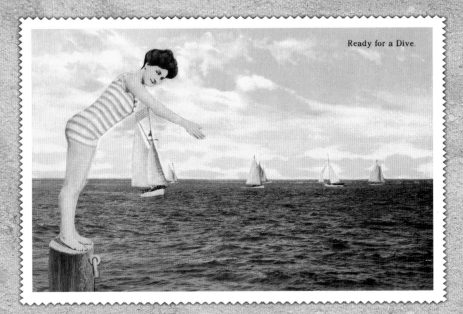

Ready for a Dive.

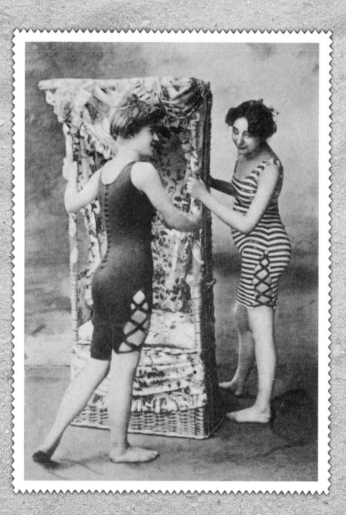

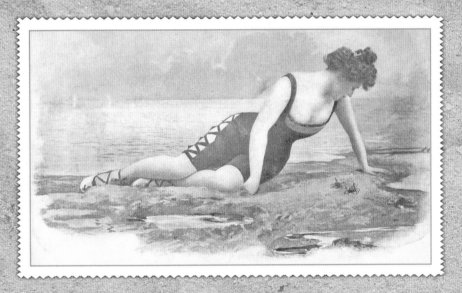

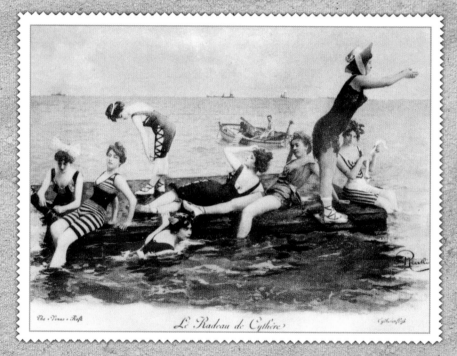

The ·Venus ·Raft   Le Radeau de Cythère   Cythère Nº6

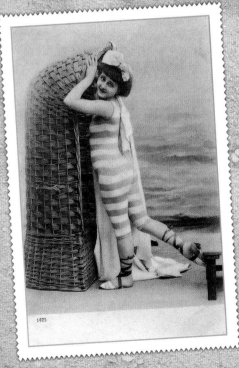

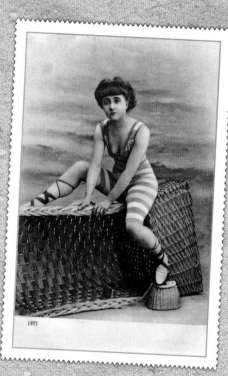

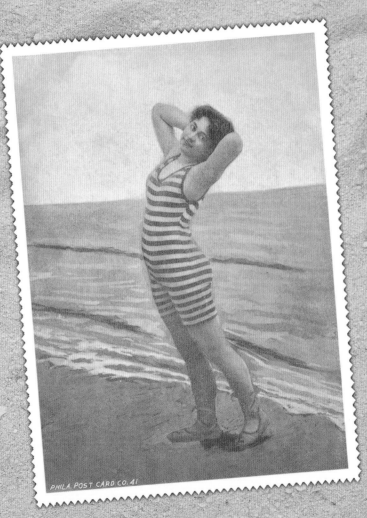

PHILA. POST CARD CO. 41

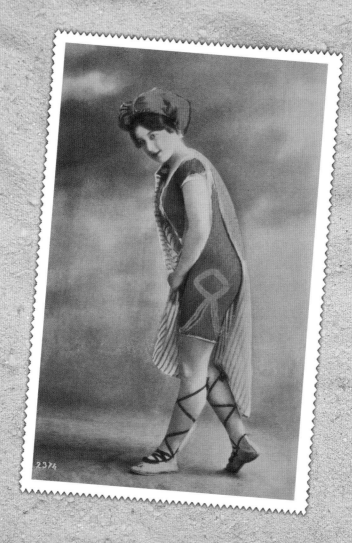

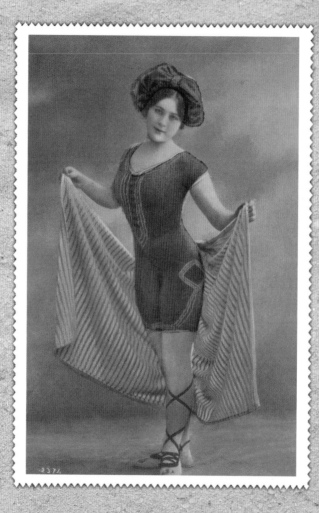

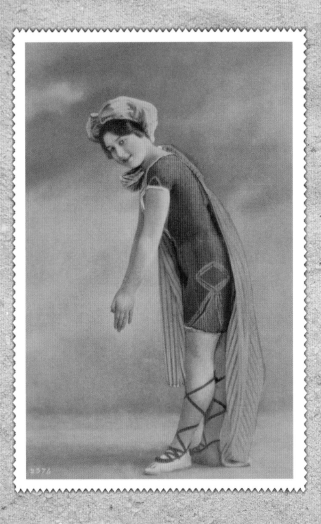

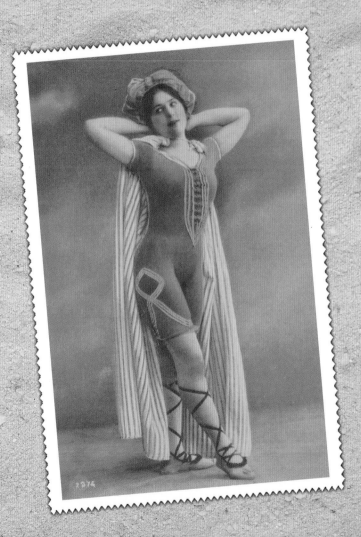

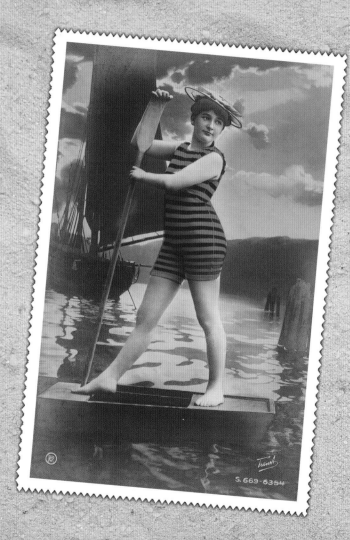

S. 669-6354

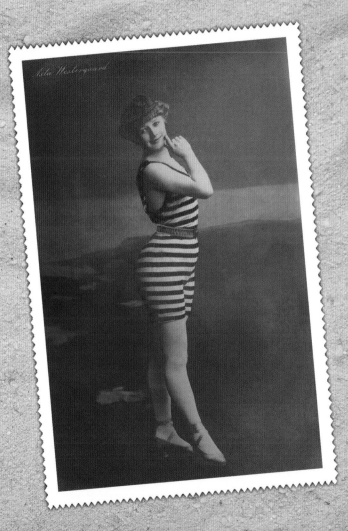

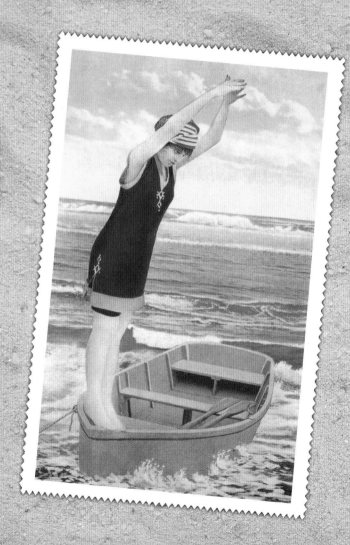

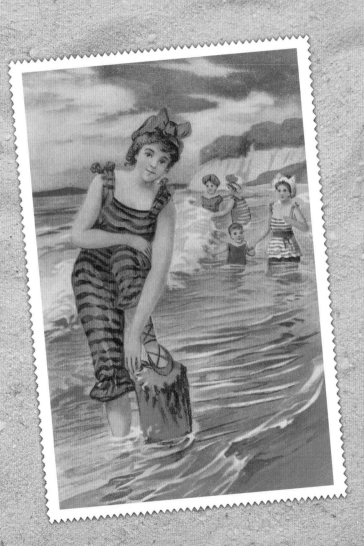

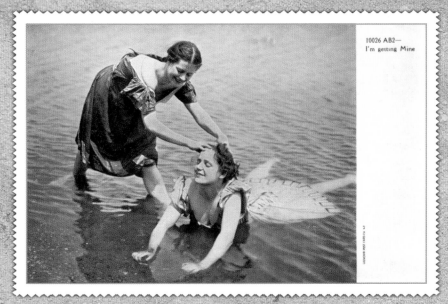

10026 AB2—
I'm getting Mine

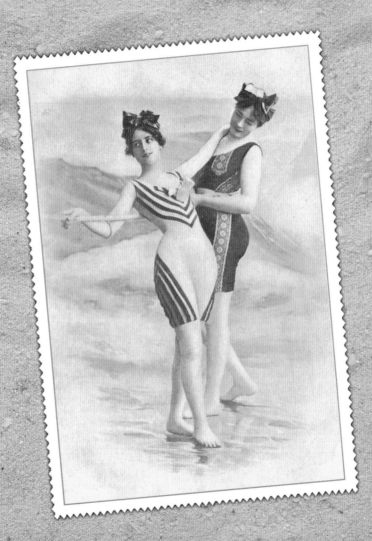

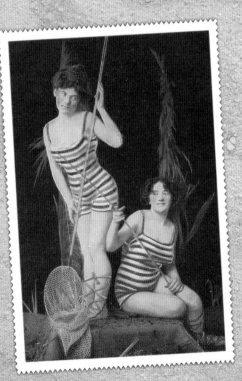
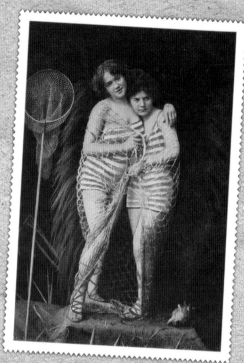

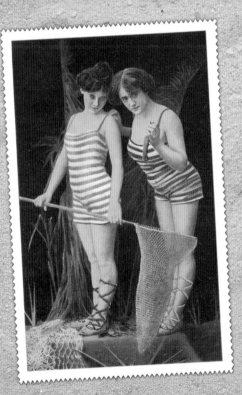
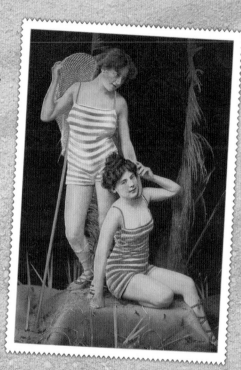

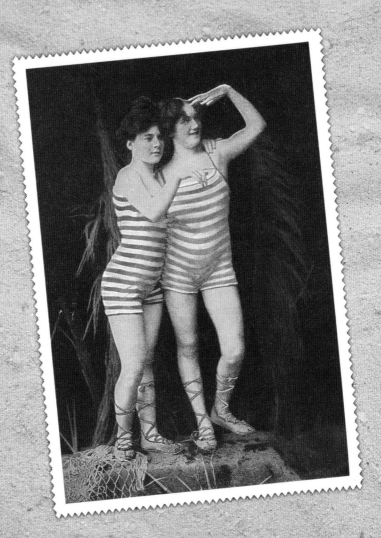

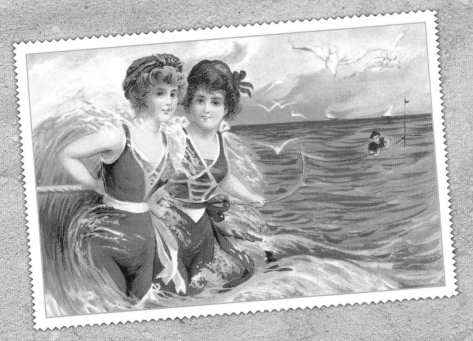

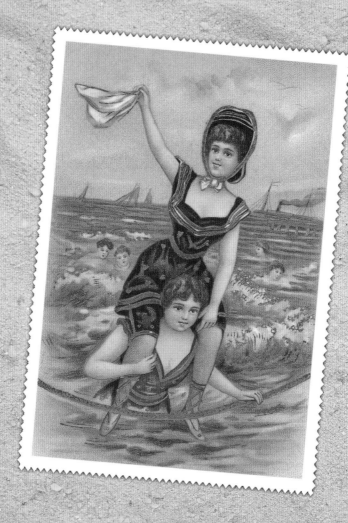

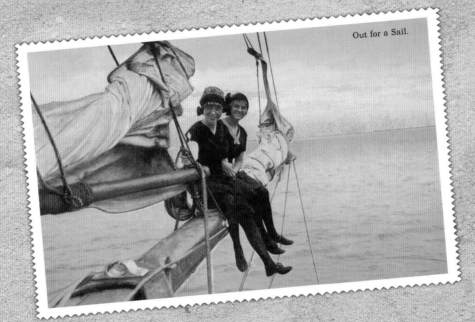

Out for a Sail.

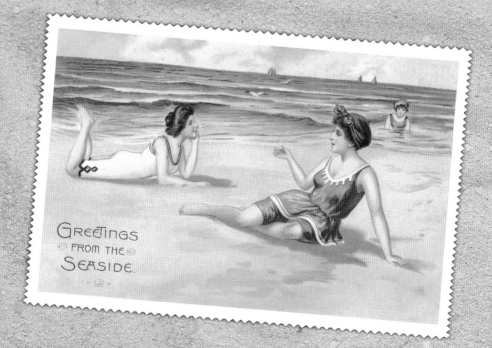

GREETINGS
FROM THE
SEASIDE.

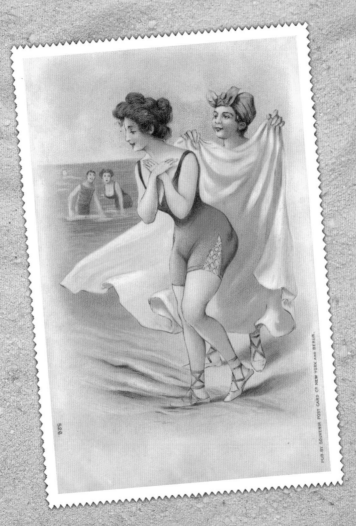

526

PUB. BY SOUVENIR POST CARD CO. NEW YORK AND BERLIN.

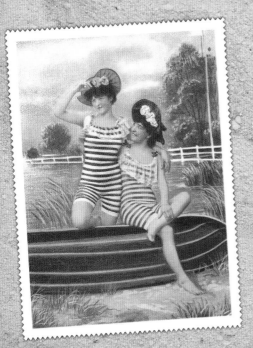
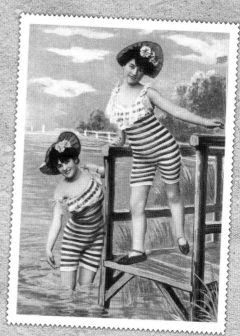

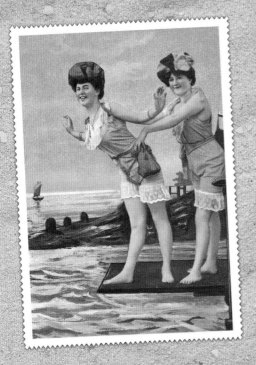
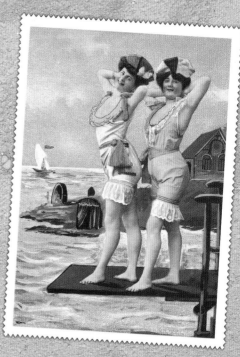

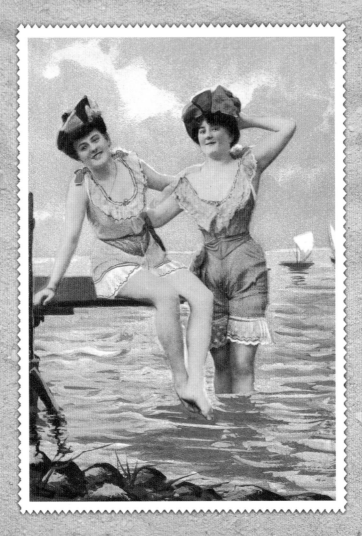

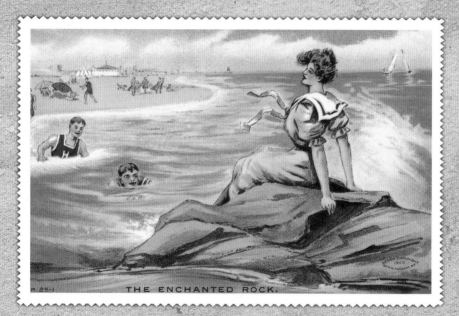

THE ENCHANTED ROCK.

In the good old summer time ~

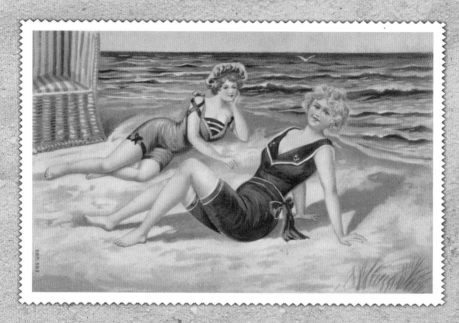

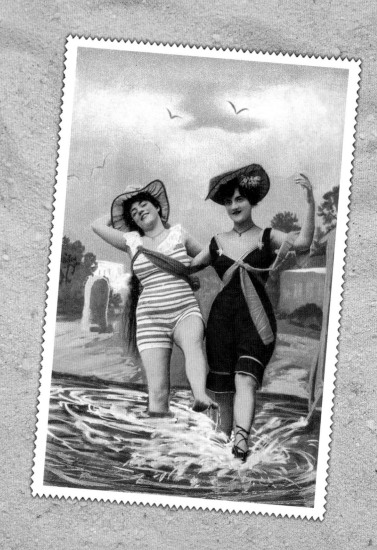

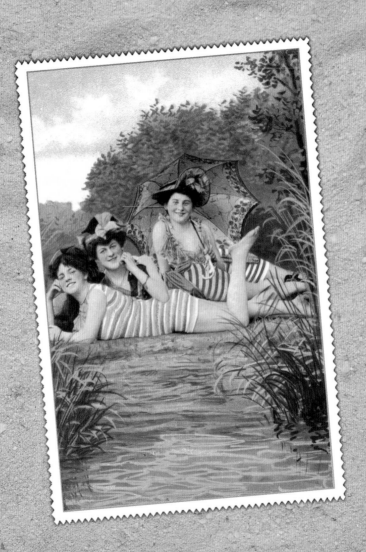

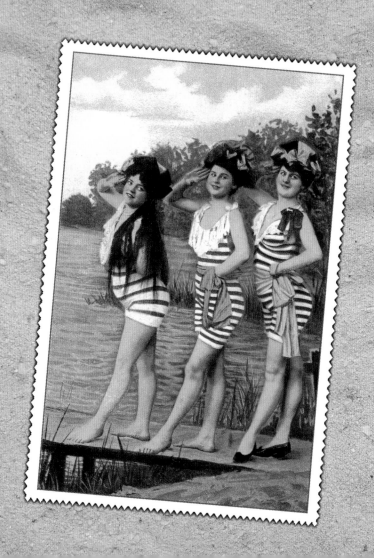

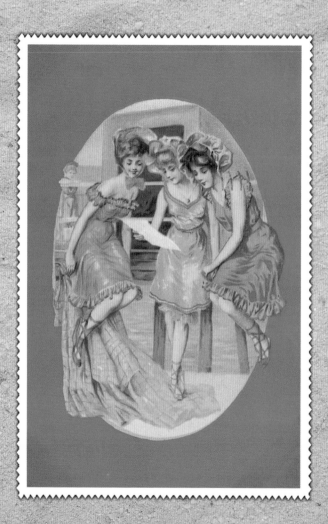

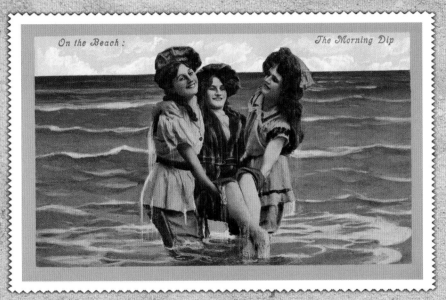

On the Beach: The Morning Dip

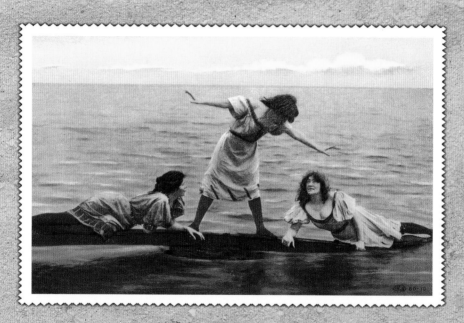

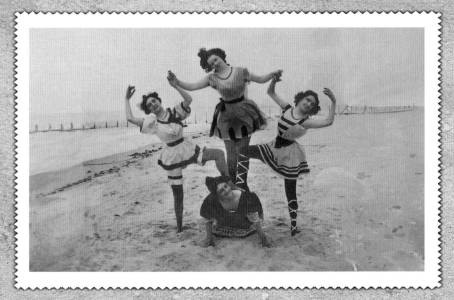

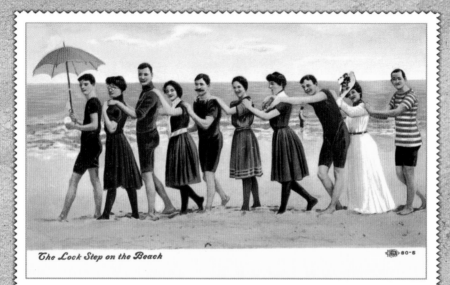

The Lock Step on the Beach

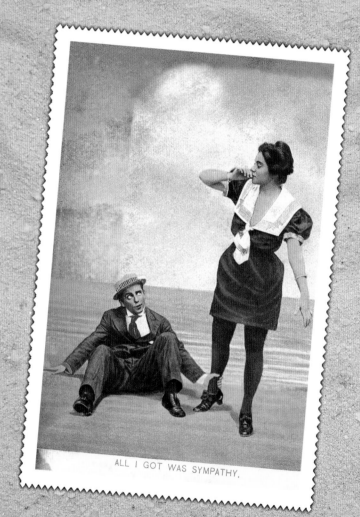

ALL I GOT WAS SYMPATHY.

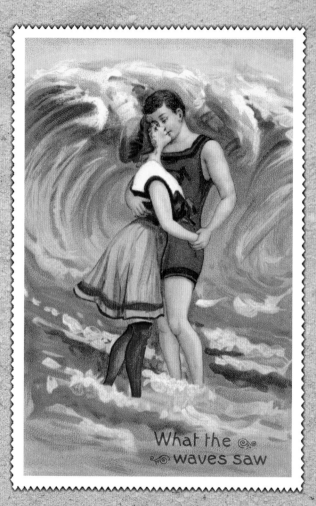

What the waves saw

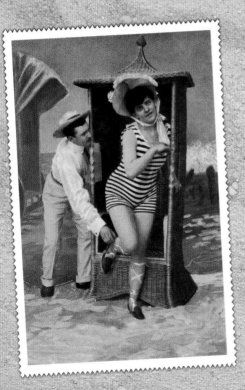
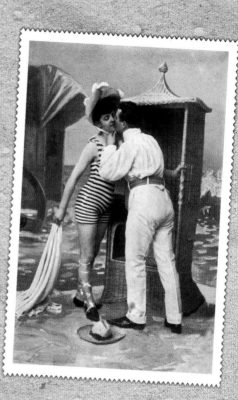

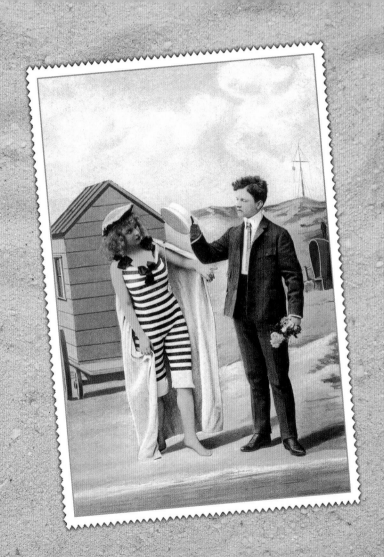

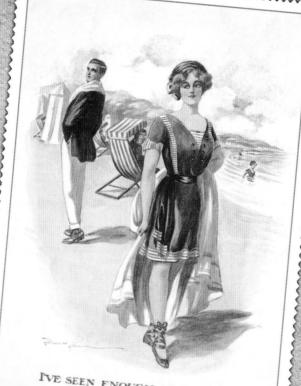

I'VE SEEN ENOUGH TO TURN
A FELLOWS HEAD

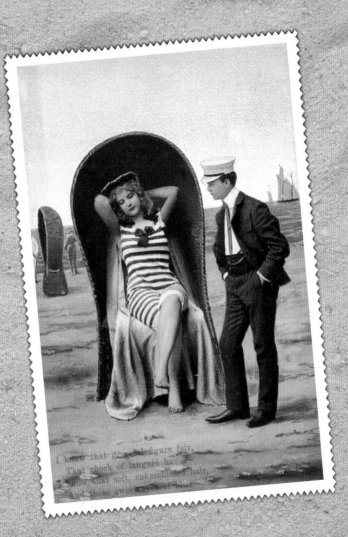

I know that graceful figure fair,
That cheek of languid hue;
I know that soft, enkerchiefed hair,
And those sweet eyes of blue.

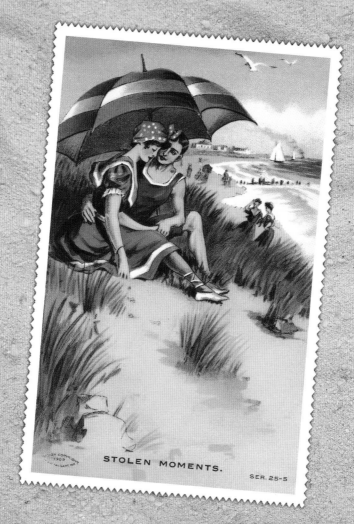

STOLEN MOMENTS.

SER. 25-5

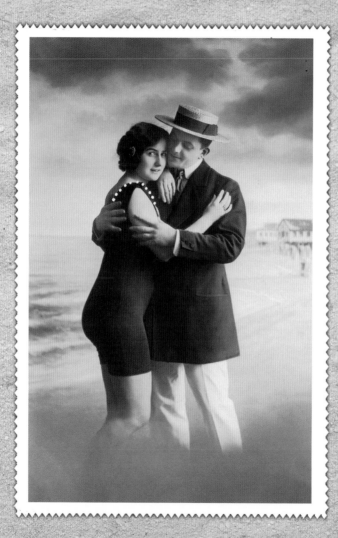

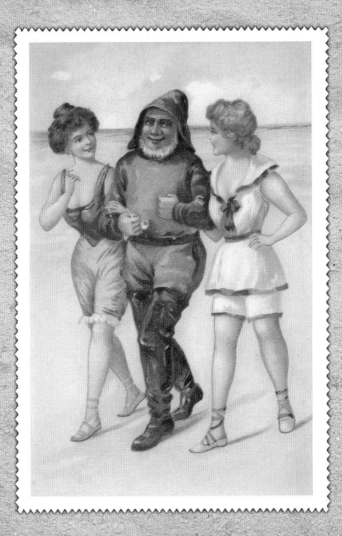

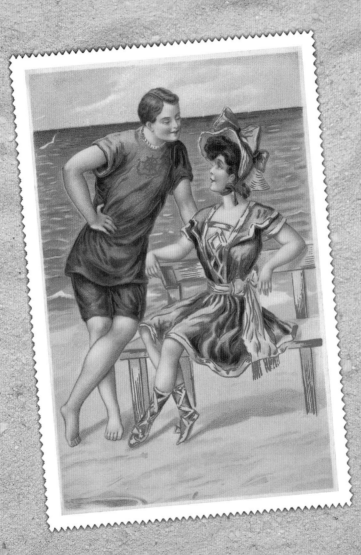

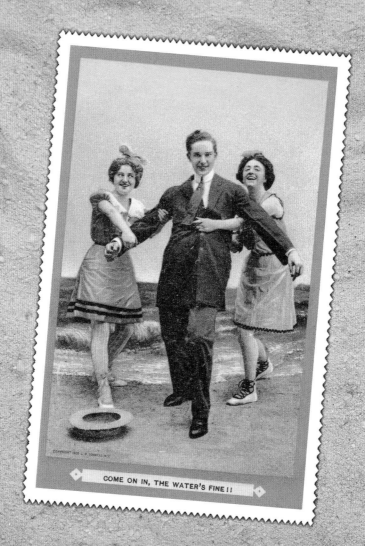

COME ON IN, THE WATER'S FINE!!

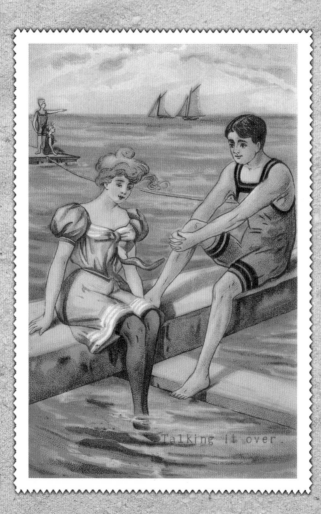

Talking it over.

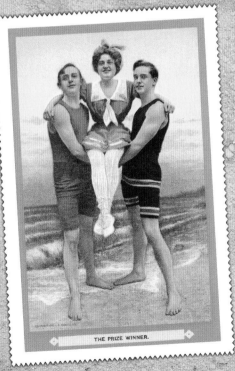

THE PRIZE WINNER.

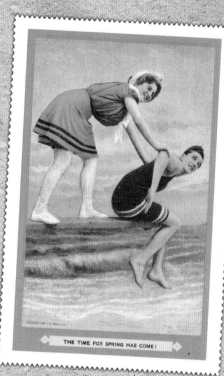

THE TIME FOR SPRING HAS COME!

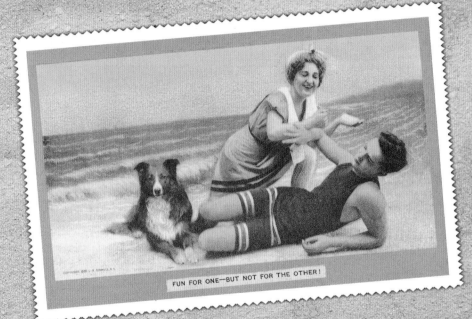

FUN FOR ONE—BUT NOT FOR THE OTHER!

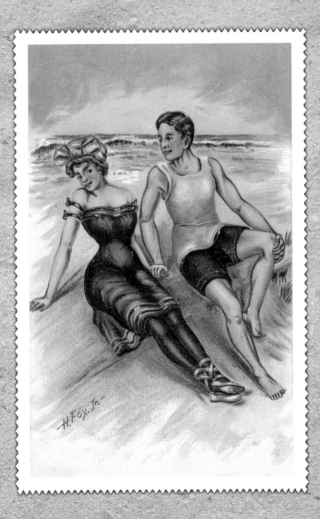

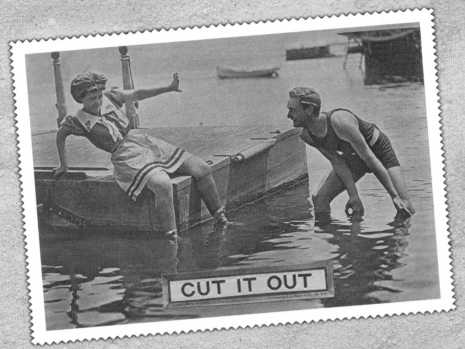

CUT IT OUT

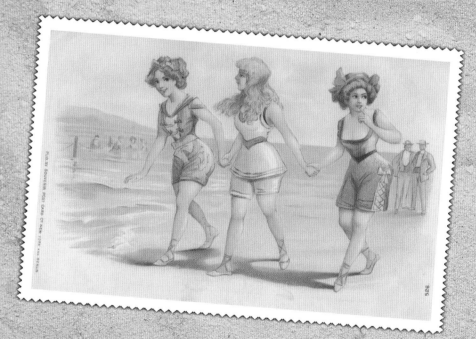

PUB. BY SOUVENIR POST CARD CO. NEW YORK AND BERLIN.

586.

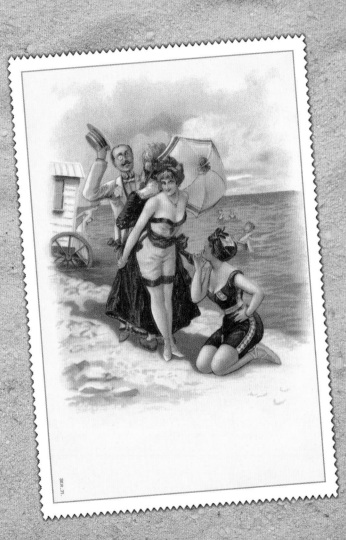

SER. 71.

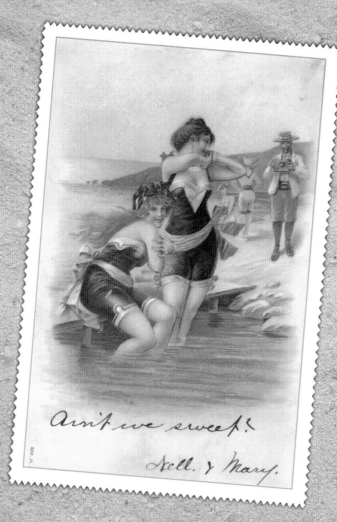

Ain't we sweet?

Nell. & Mary.

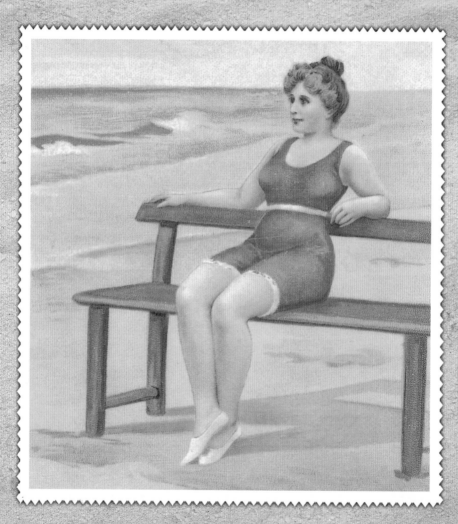